This Book Belongs to

____

____

____

Note: if using real makeup, allow page to dry completely before turning or closing. A short burst from a hair dryer can aid this process.

Name of Look _______________________   Evening ◯   Daytime ◯

Theme _______________________

Face

Moisturizer

Concealer

Foundation

Highlight/Blush

Eyes

Brows

Eyelid

Liner

Crease

Mascara

Lips

Liner

Lip Color

Gloss

Notes

Makeup

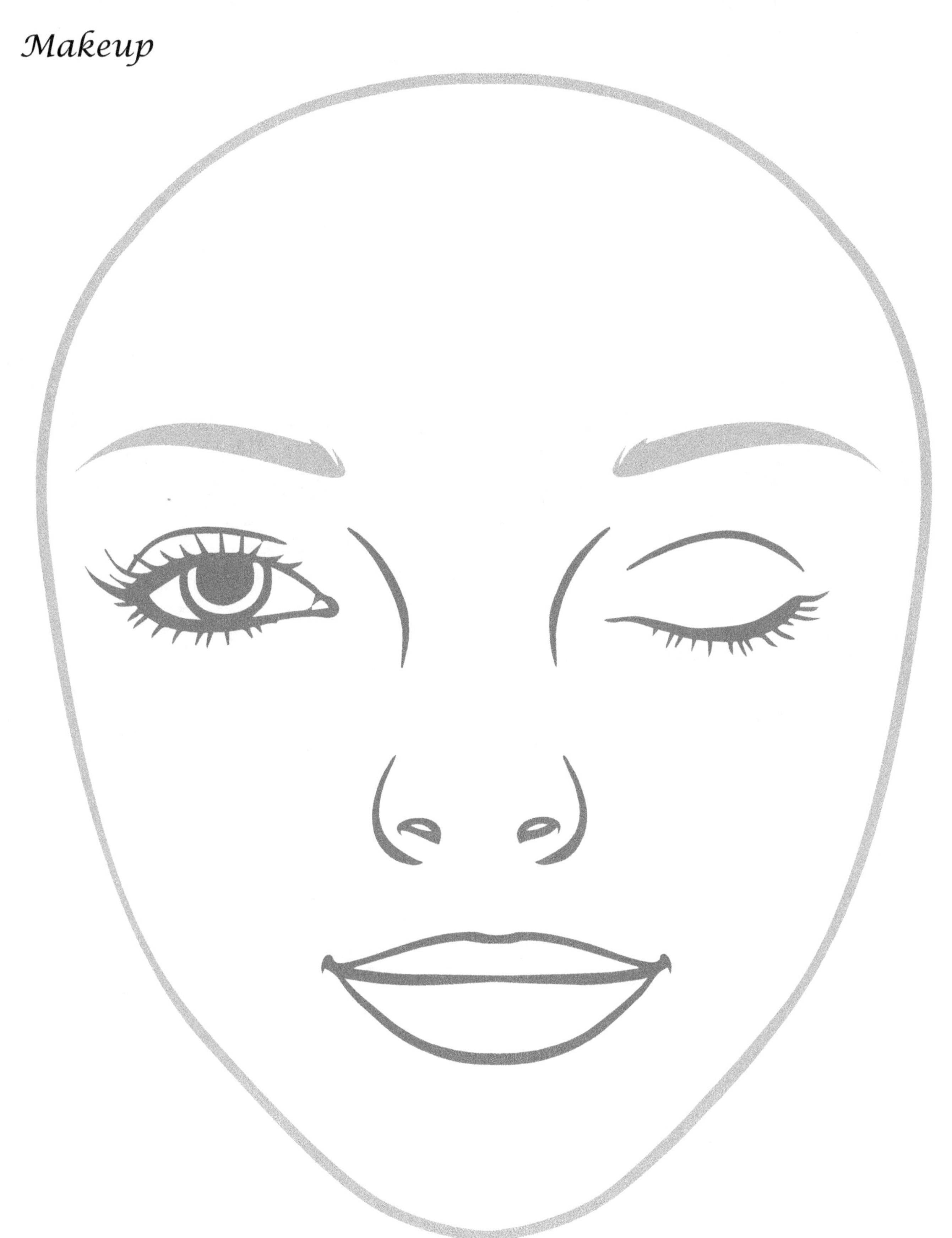

Checklist

Checklist

Name of Look ____ Evening ◯ Daytime ◯

Theme ____

Face	Eyes	Lips
Moisturizer	Brows	Liner
Concealer	Eyelid	Lip Color
Foundation	Liner	Gloss
Highlight/Blush	Crease	
	Mascara	

Notes

Makeup

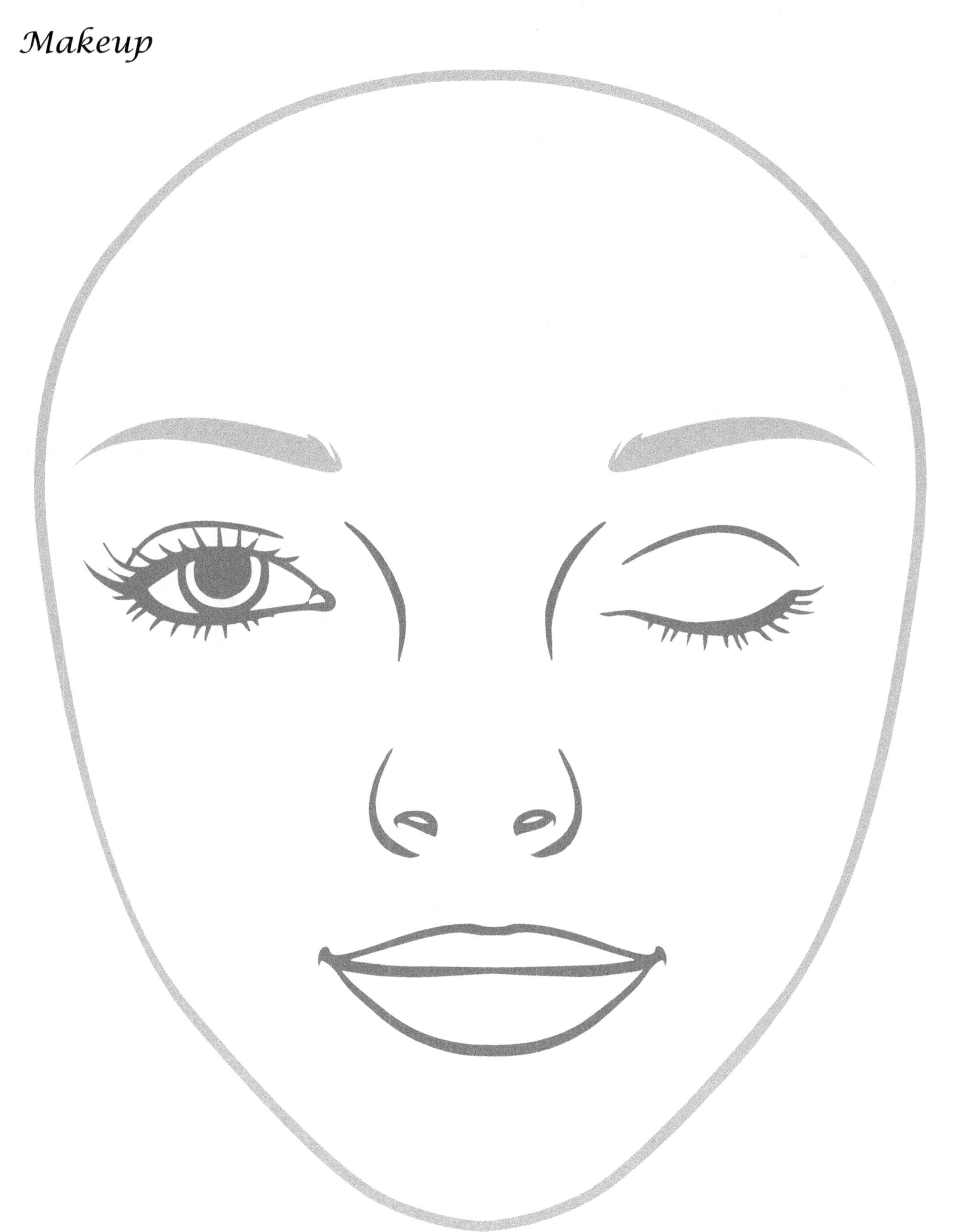

Checklist

Checklist

Name of Look _______________________   **Evening** ◯   **Daytime** ◯

Theme ____

Face

Moisturizer

Concealer

Foundation

Highlight/Blush

Eyes

Brows

Eyelid

Liner

Crease

Mascara

Lips

Liner

Lip Color

Gloss

Notes

Makeup

Checklist

Checklist

Face

Moisturizer

Concealer

Foundation

Highlight/Blush

Eyes

Brows

Eyelid

Liner

Crease

Mascara

Lips

Liner

Lip Color

Gloss

Notes

Makeup

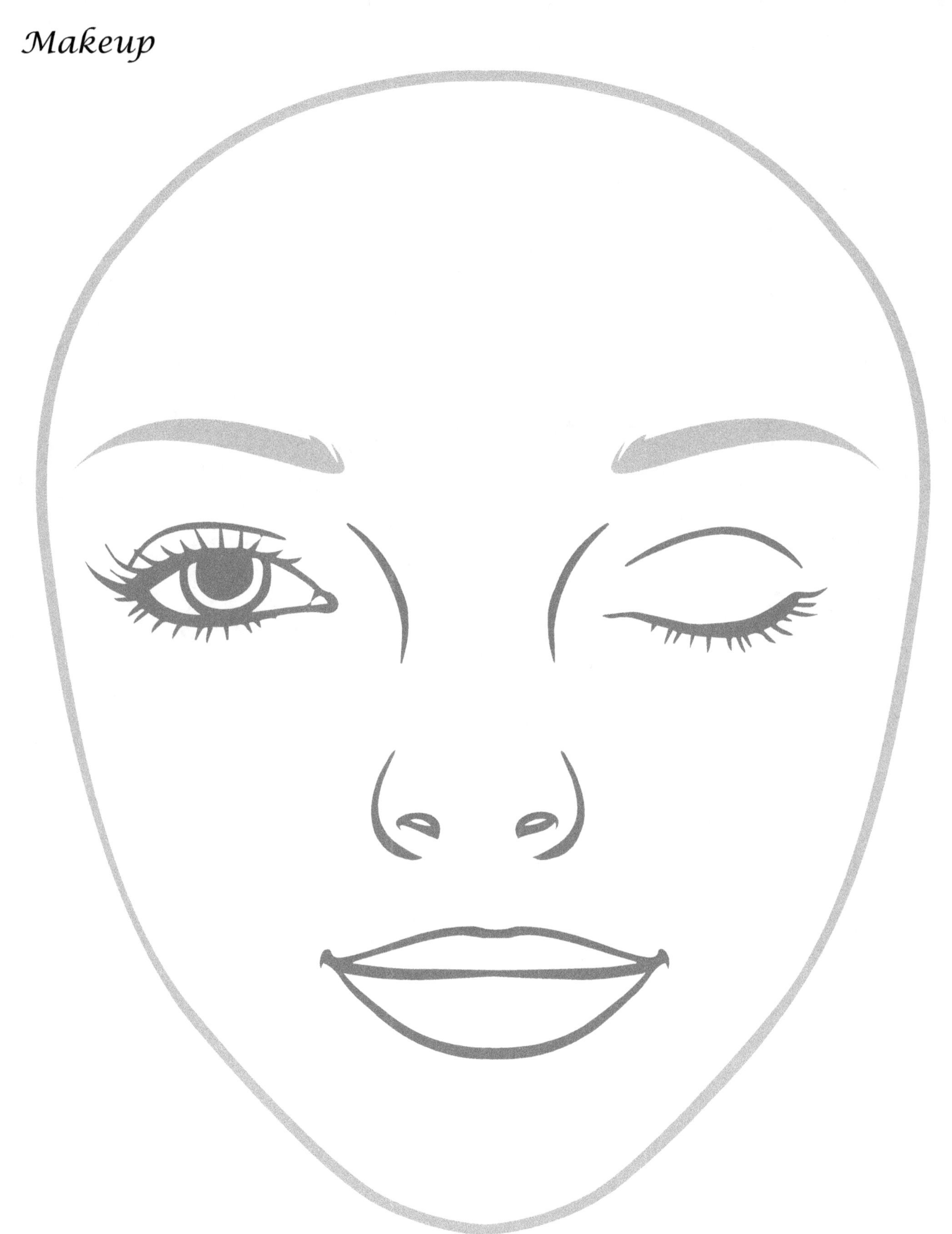

Checklist

Checklist

Name of Look _______________________________   **Evening** ◯   **Daytime** ◯

Theme ____

Face

Moisturizer

Concealer

Foundation

Highlight/Blush

Eyes

Brows

Eyelid

Liner

Crease

Mascara

Lips

Liner

Lip Color

Gloss

Notes

Makeup

Checklist

Checklist

Name of Look ___________________________   **Evening** ◯   **Daytime** ◯

Theme ___________________________

Face

Moisturizer

Concealer

Foundation

Highlight/Blush

Eyes

Brows

Eyelid

Liner

Crease

Mascara

Lips

Liner

Lip Color

Gloss

Notes

Makeup

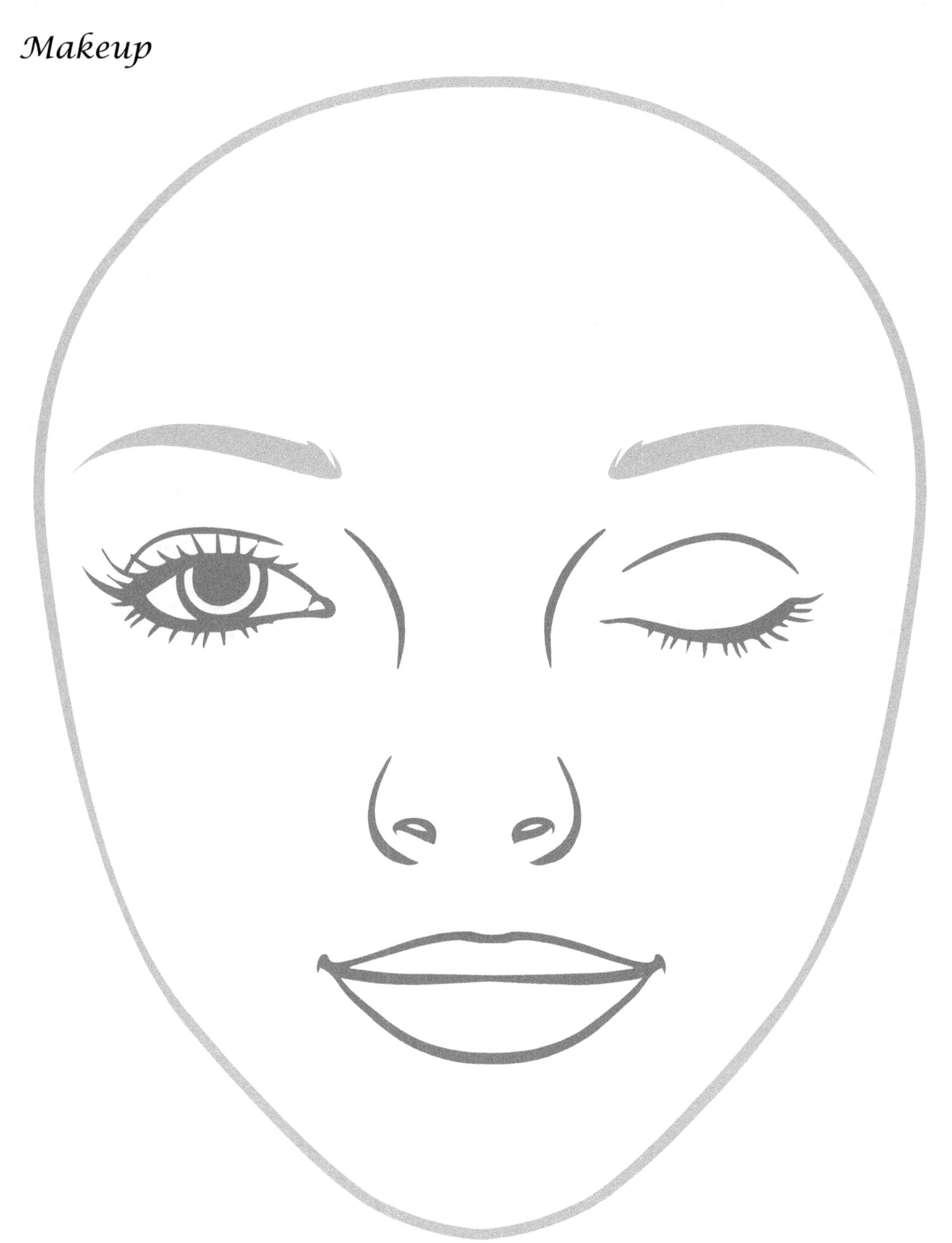

Checklist

Checklist

Name of Look _______________________   **Evening** ◯   **Daytime** ◯

Theme _______________________

Face

Moisturizer

Concealer

Foundation

Highlight/Blush

Eyes

Brows

Eyelid

Liner

Crease

Mascara

Lips

Liner

Lip Color

Gloss

Notes

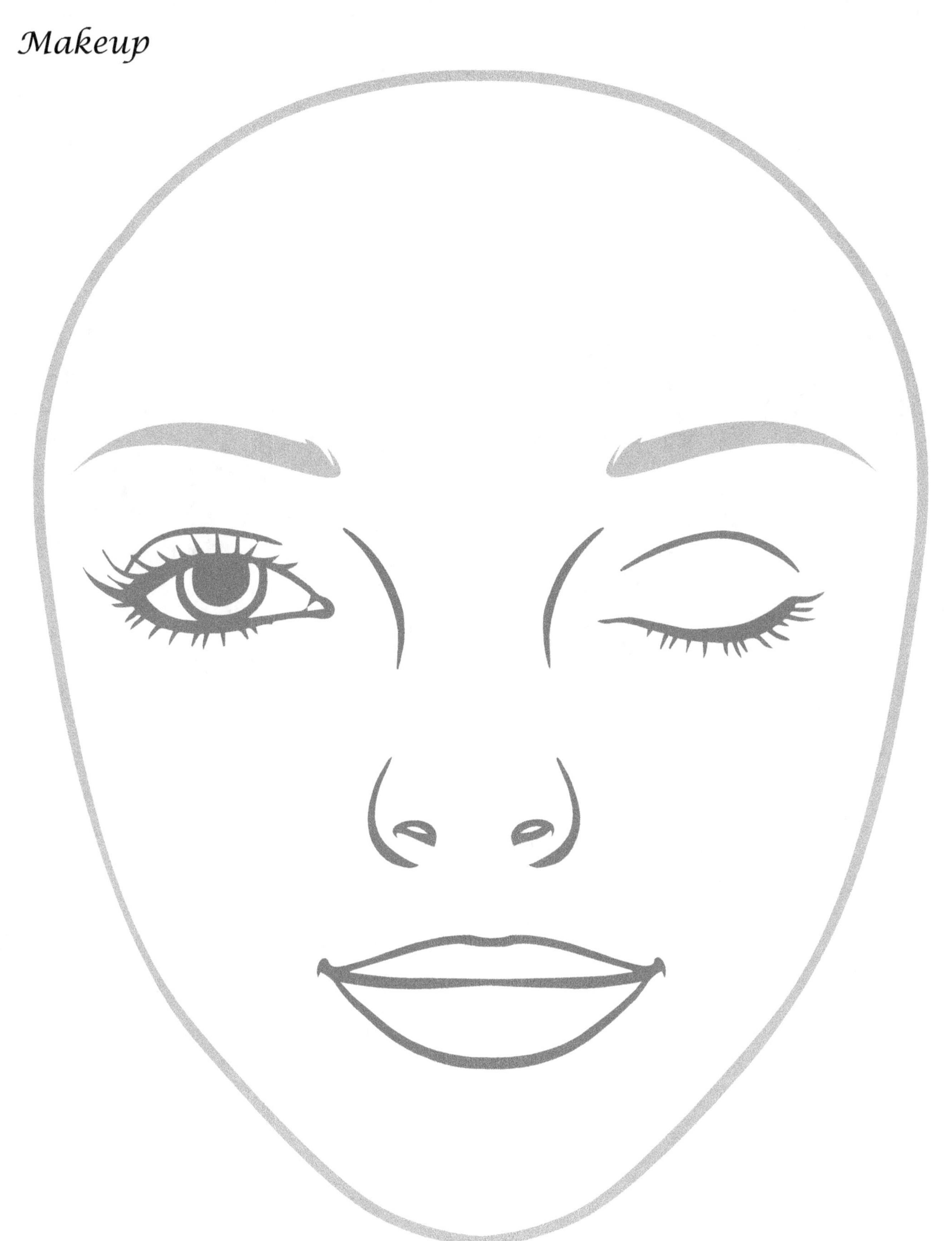

Makeup

Checklist

Checklist

Face

Moisturizer

Concealer

Foundation

Highlight/Blush

Eyes

Brows

Eyelid

Liner

Crease

Mascara

Lips

Liner

Lip Color

Gloss

Notes

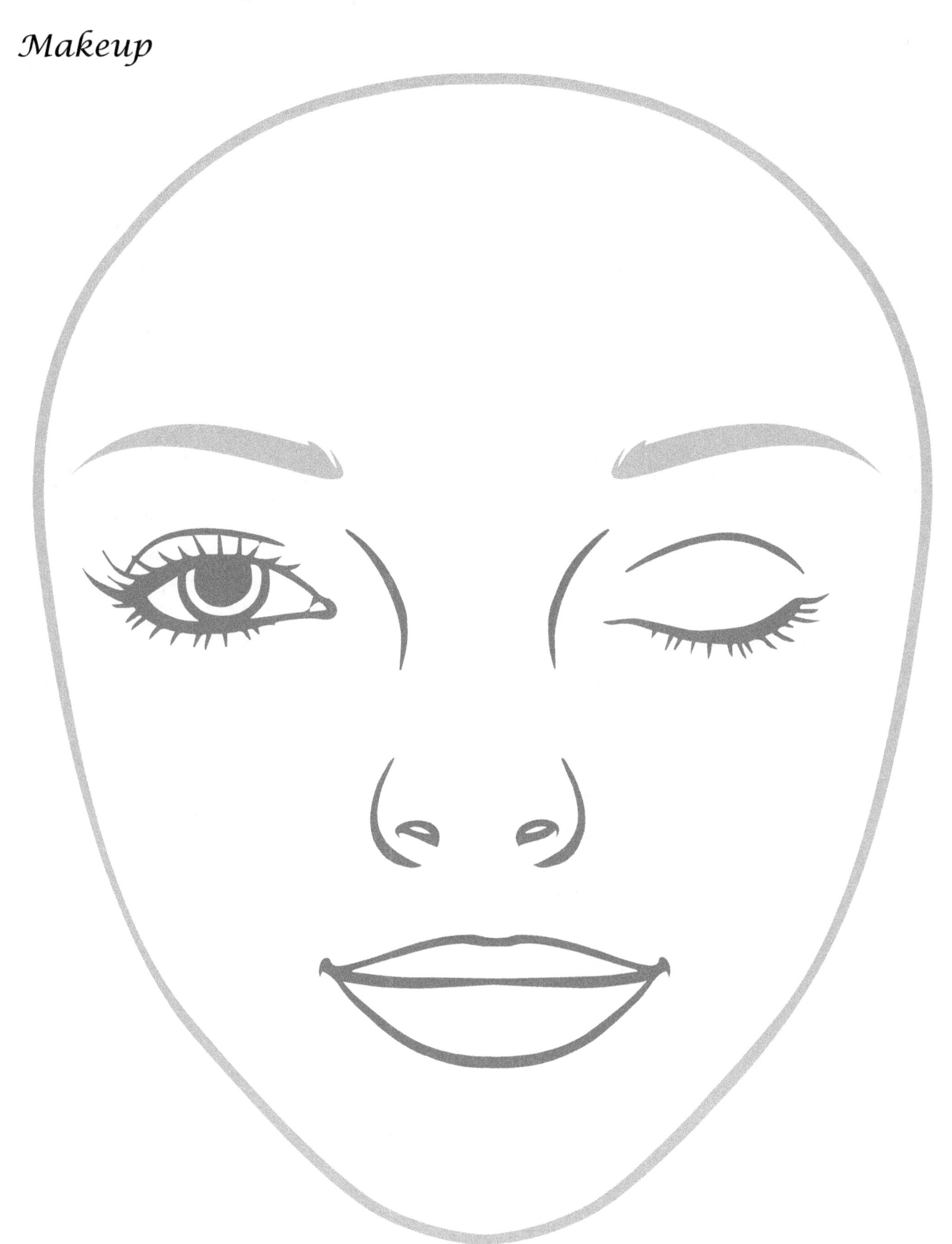
Makeup

Checklist

Checklist

Name of Look ___________________________ **Evening** ◯ **Daytime** ◯

Theme ___________________________

Face

Moisturizer

Concealer

Foundation

Highlight/Blush

Eyes

Brows

Eyelid

Liner

Crease

Mascara

Lips

Liner

Lip Color

Gloss

Notes

Makeup

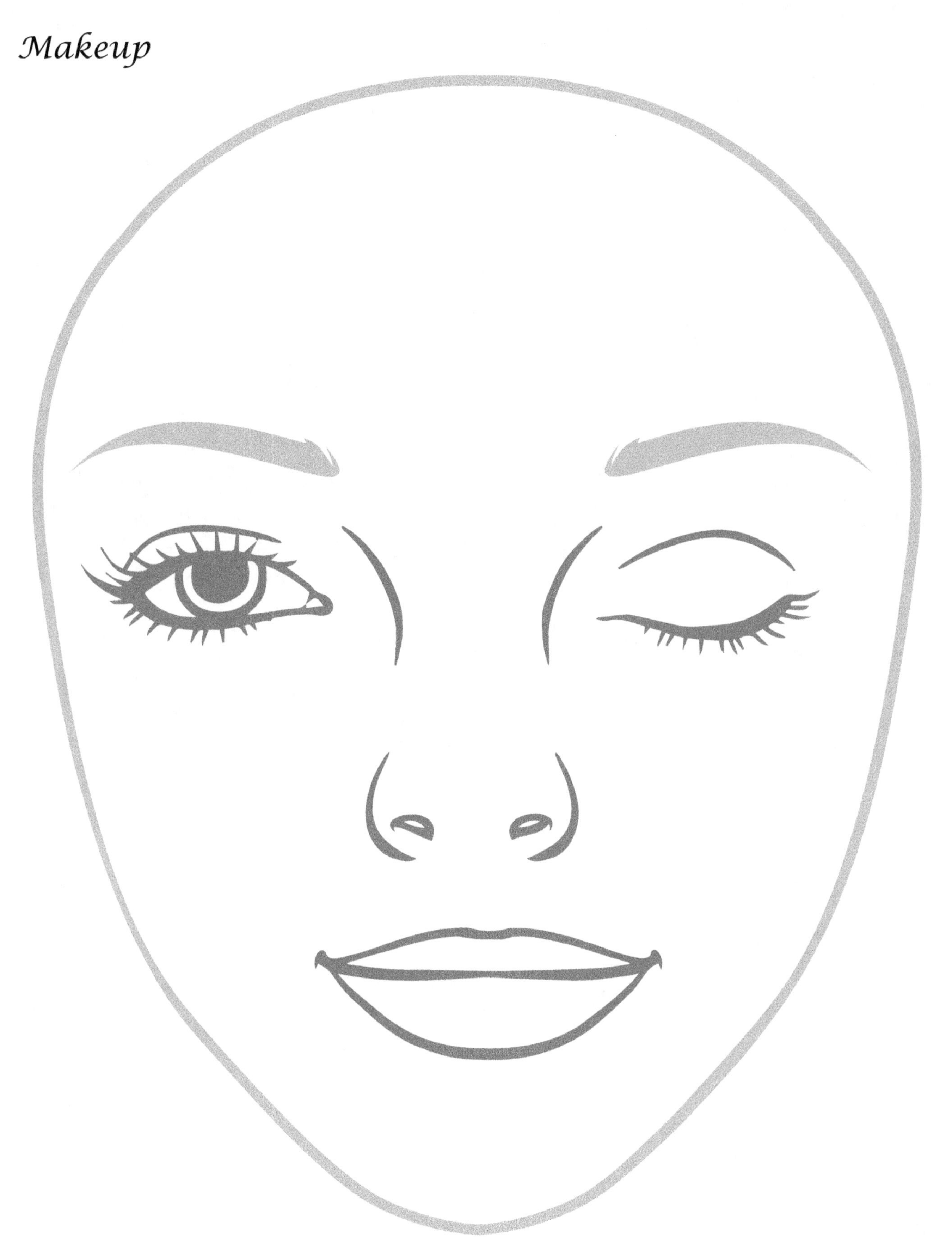

Checklist

Checklist

Name of Look _______________________ **Evening** ◯   **Daytime** ◯

Theme _______________________

Face

Moisturizer

Concealer

Foundation

Highlight/Blush

Eyes

Brows

Eyelid

Liner

Crease

Mascara

Lips

Liner

Lip Color

Gloss

Notes

Makeup

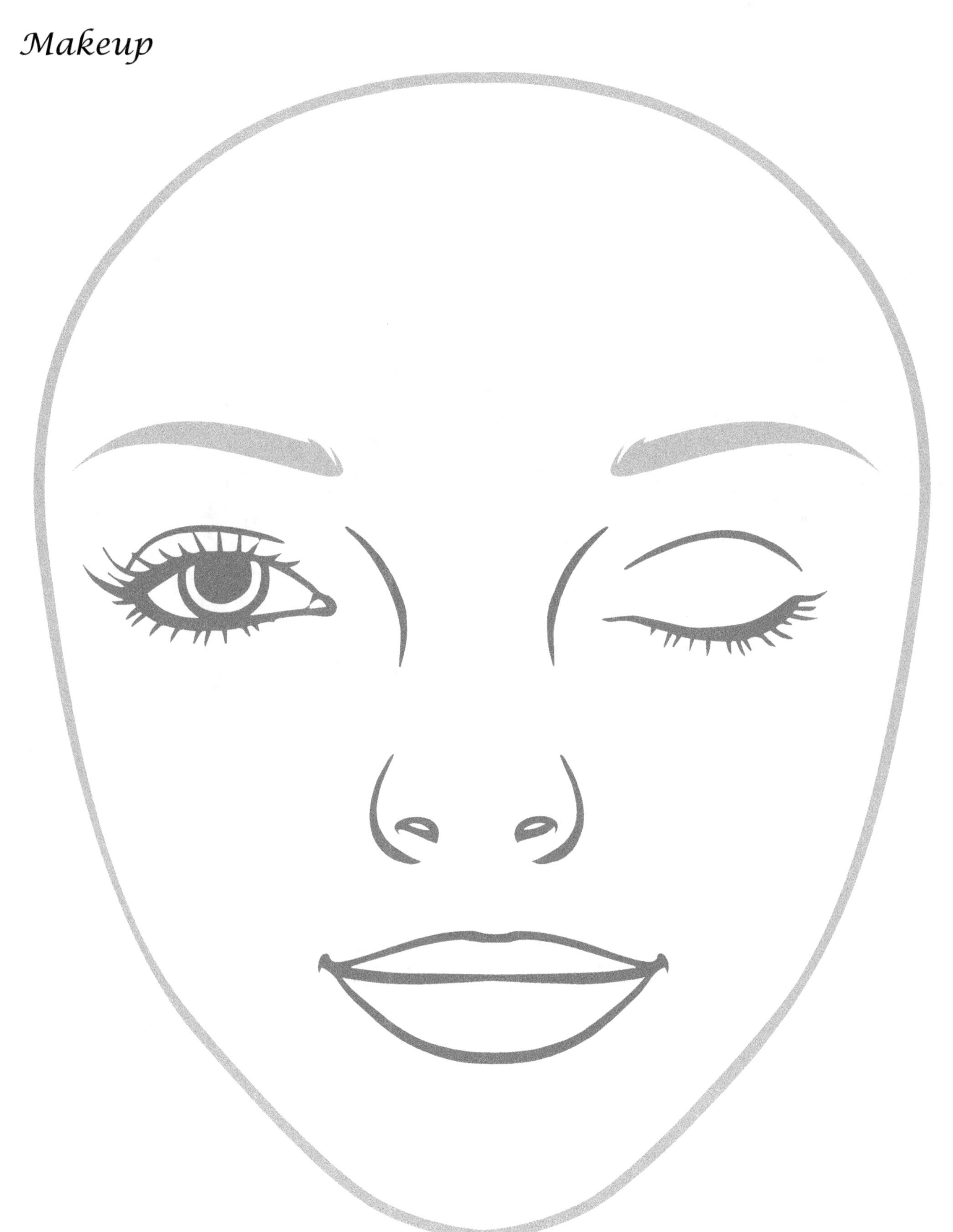

Checklist

Checklist

Name of Look ______________________ **Evening** ◯ **Daytime** ◯

Theme ____

Face	**Eyes**	**Lips**
Moisturizer	Brows	Liner
Concealer	Eyelid	Lip Color
Foundation	Liner	Gloss
Highlight/Blush	Crease	
	Mascara	

Notes

Makeup

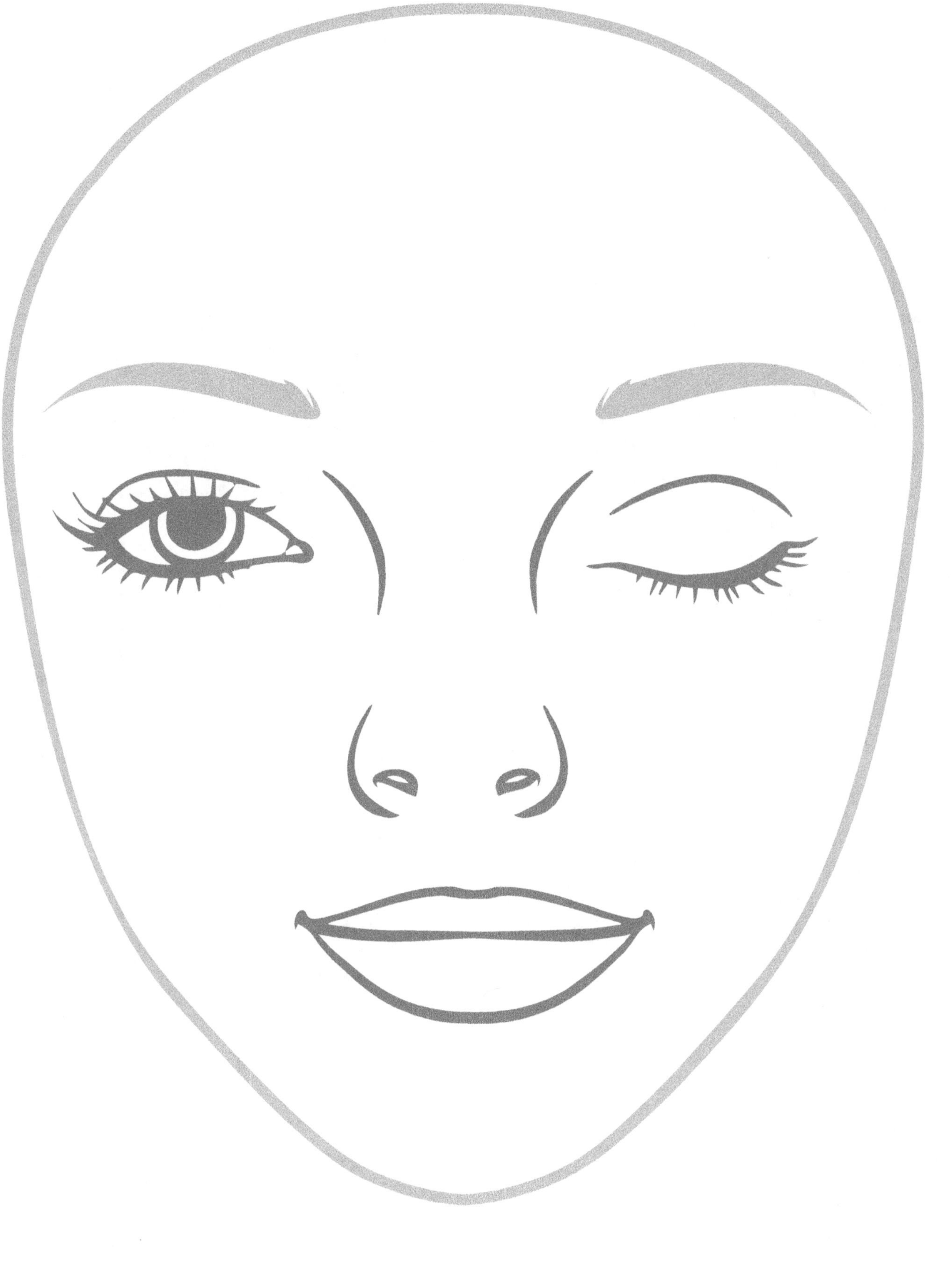

Checklist

Checklist

Name of Look _________________________________   **Evening** ◯   **Daytime** ◯

Theme ____

Face	**Eyes**	**Lips**
Moisturizer	Brows	Liner
Concealer	Eyelid	Lip Color
Foundation	Liner	Gloss
Highlight/Blush	Crease	
	Mascara	

Notes

Makeup

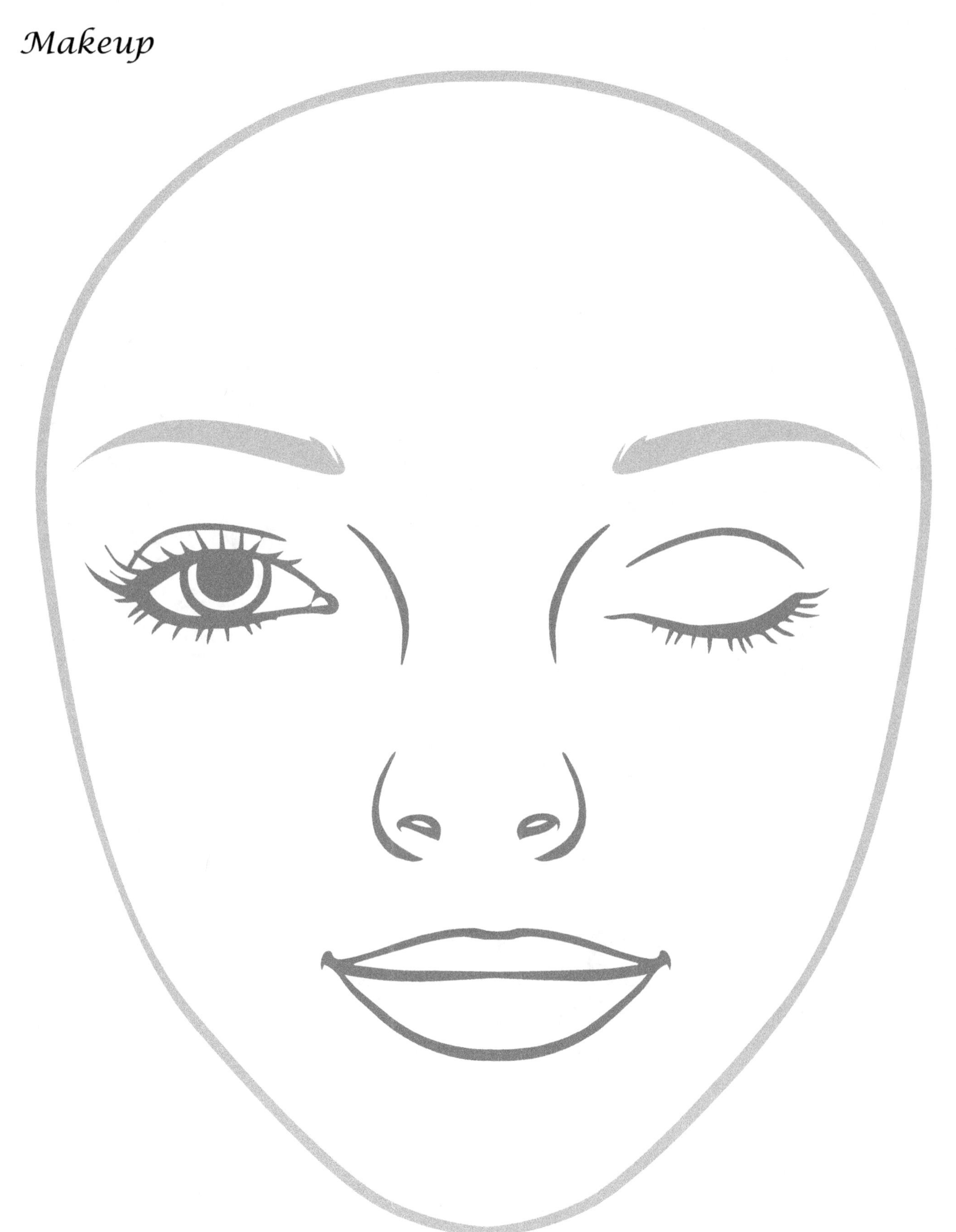

Checklist

Checklist

Name of Look _______________________ **Evening** ◯ **Daytime** ◯

Theme _______________________

Face

Moisturizer

Concealer

Foundation

Highlight/Blush

Eyes

Brows

Eyelid

Liner

Crease

Mascara

Lips

Liner

Lip Color

Gloss

Notes

Makeup

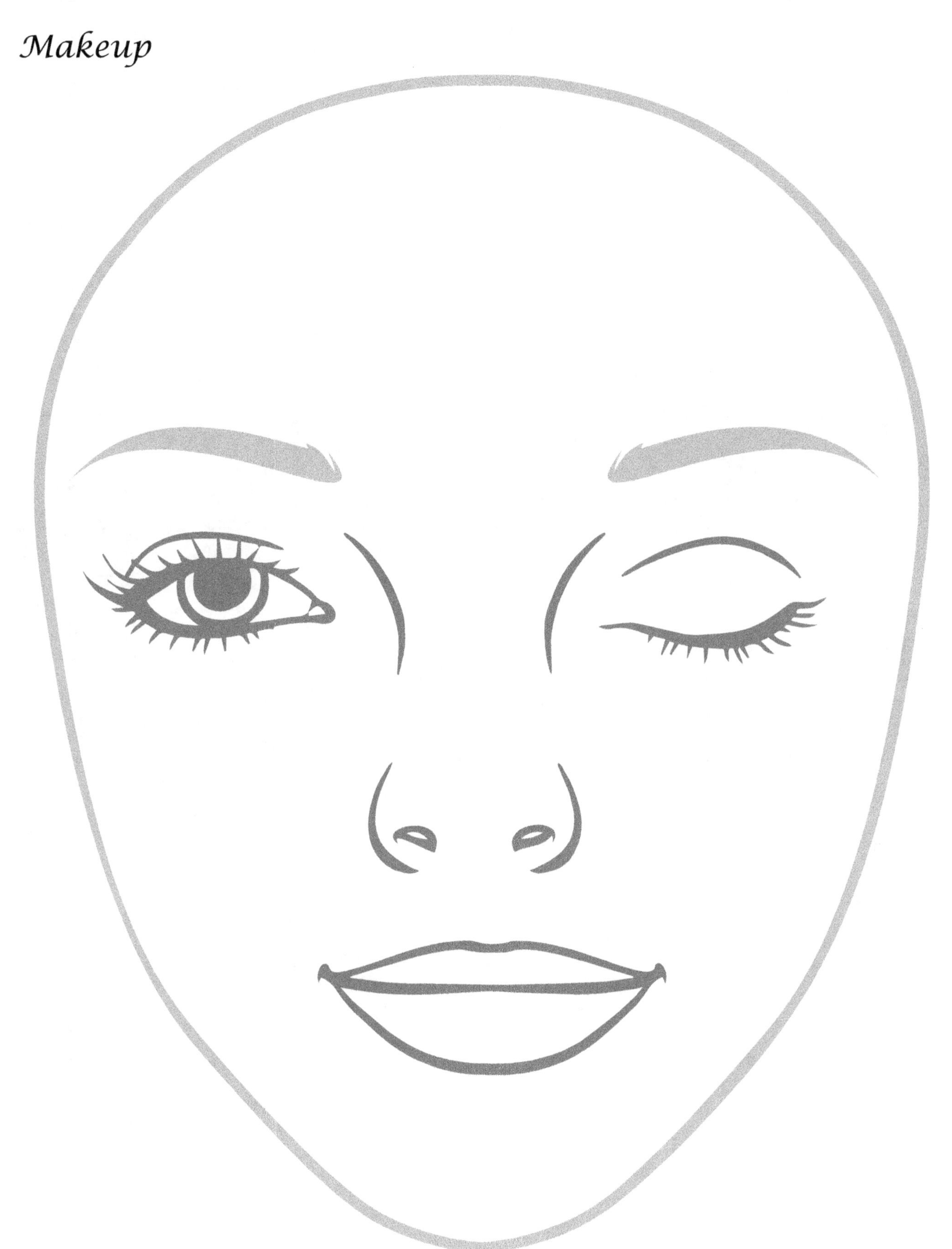

Checklist

Checklist

Name of Look ______________________   **Evening** ◯   **Daytime** ◯

Theme ______________________

Face	**Eyes**	**Lips**
Moisturizer	Brows	Liner
Concealer	Eyelid	Lip Color
Foundation	Liner	Gloss
Highlight/Blush	Crease	
	Mascara	

Notes

Makeup

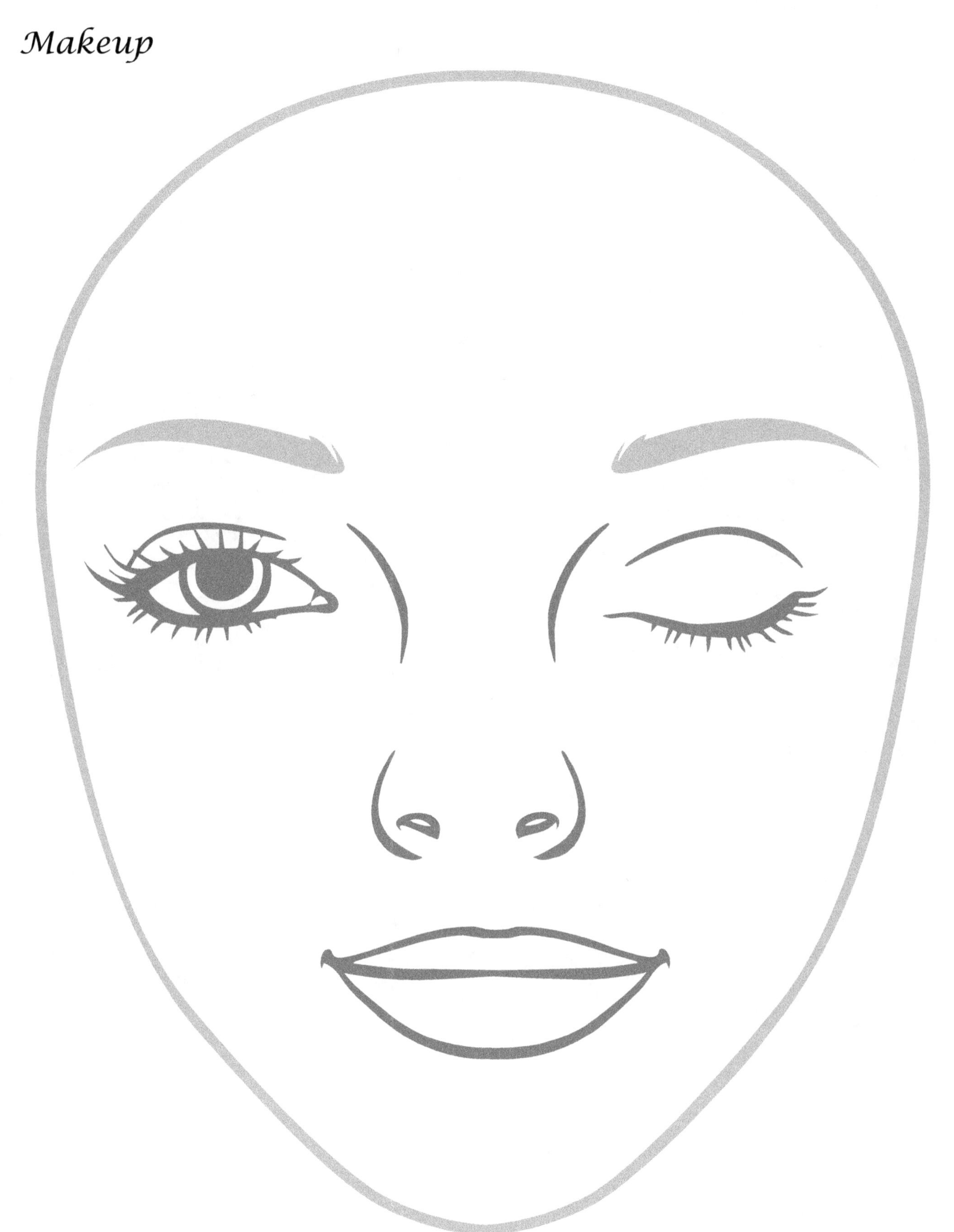

Checklist

Checklist

Name of Look ______________________________   **Evening** ◯   **Daytime** ◯

Theme ____

Face	**Eyes**	**Lips**
Moisturizer	Brows	Liner
Concealer	Eyelid	Lip Color
Foundation	Liner	Gloss
Highlight/Blush	Crease	
	Mascara	

Notes

Makeup

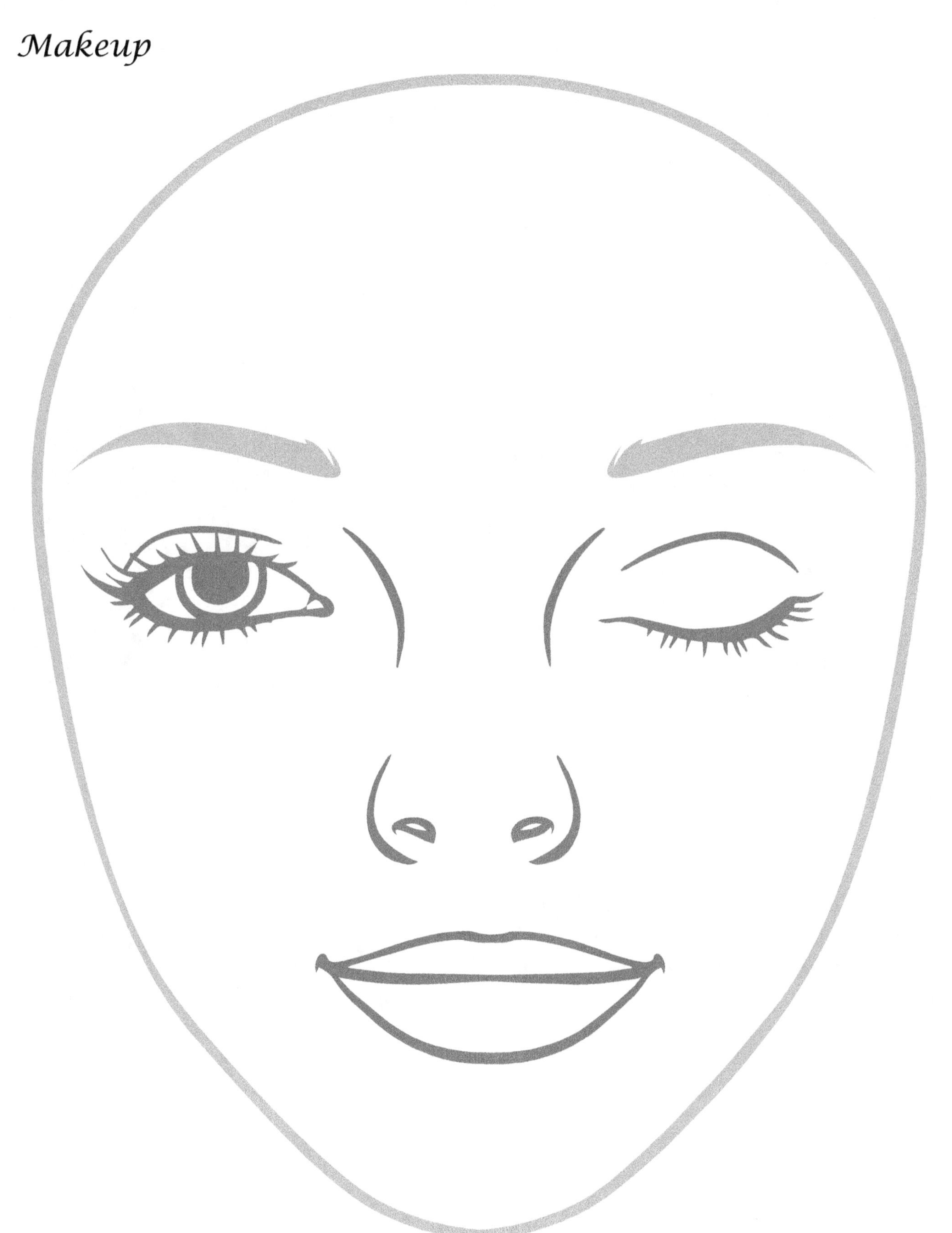

Checklist

Checklist

Name of Look _______________________   **Evening** ◯   **Daytime** ◯

Theme _______________________

Face

Moisturizer

Concealer

Foundation

Highlight/Blush

Eyes

Brows

Eyelid

Liner

Crease

Mascara

Lips

Liner

Lip Color

Gloss

Notes

Makeup

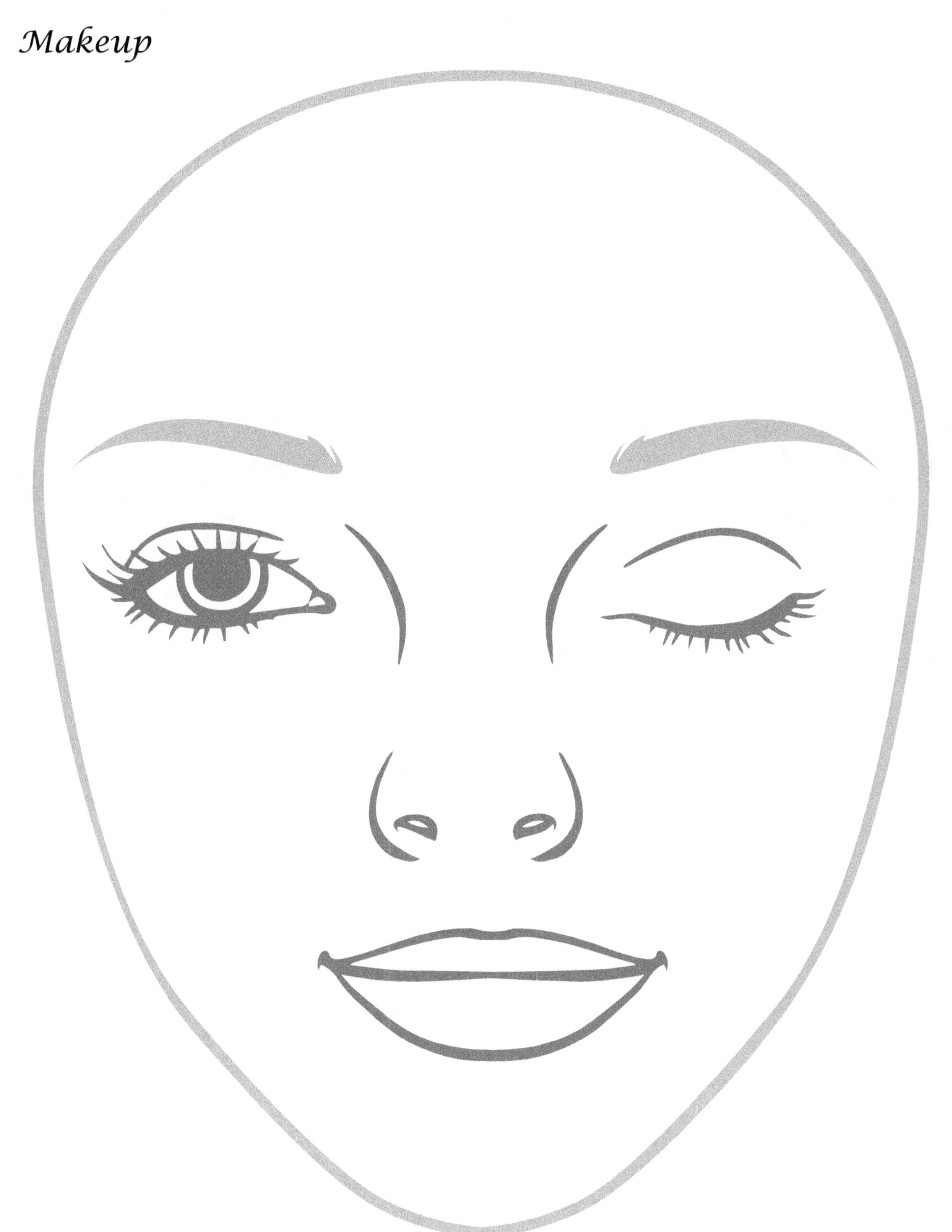

Checklist

Checklist

Name of Look _______________________ **Evening** ○ **Daytime** ○

Theme ____

Face

Moisturizer

Concealer

Foundation

Highlight/Blush

Eyes

Brows

Eyelid

Liner

Crease

Mascara

Lips

Liner

Lip Color

Gloss

Notes

Makeup

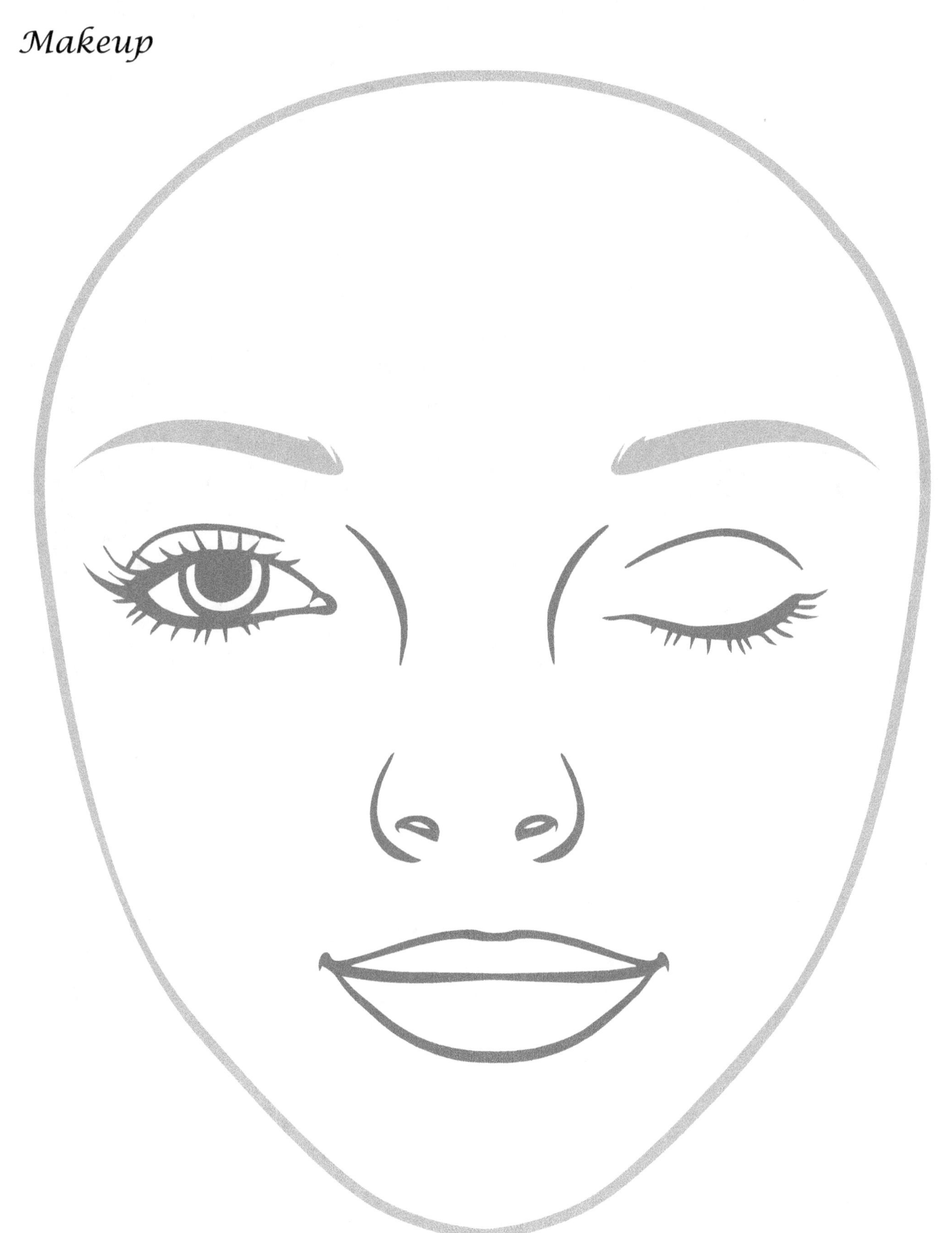

Checklist

Checklist

Name of Look ______________________________   **Evening** ◯   **Daytime** ◯

Theme ______________________________

Face	**Eyes**	**Lips**
Moisturizer	Brows	Liner
Concealer	Eyelid	Lip Color
Foundation	Liner	Gloss
Highlight/Blush	Crease	
	Mascara	

Notes

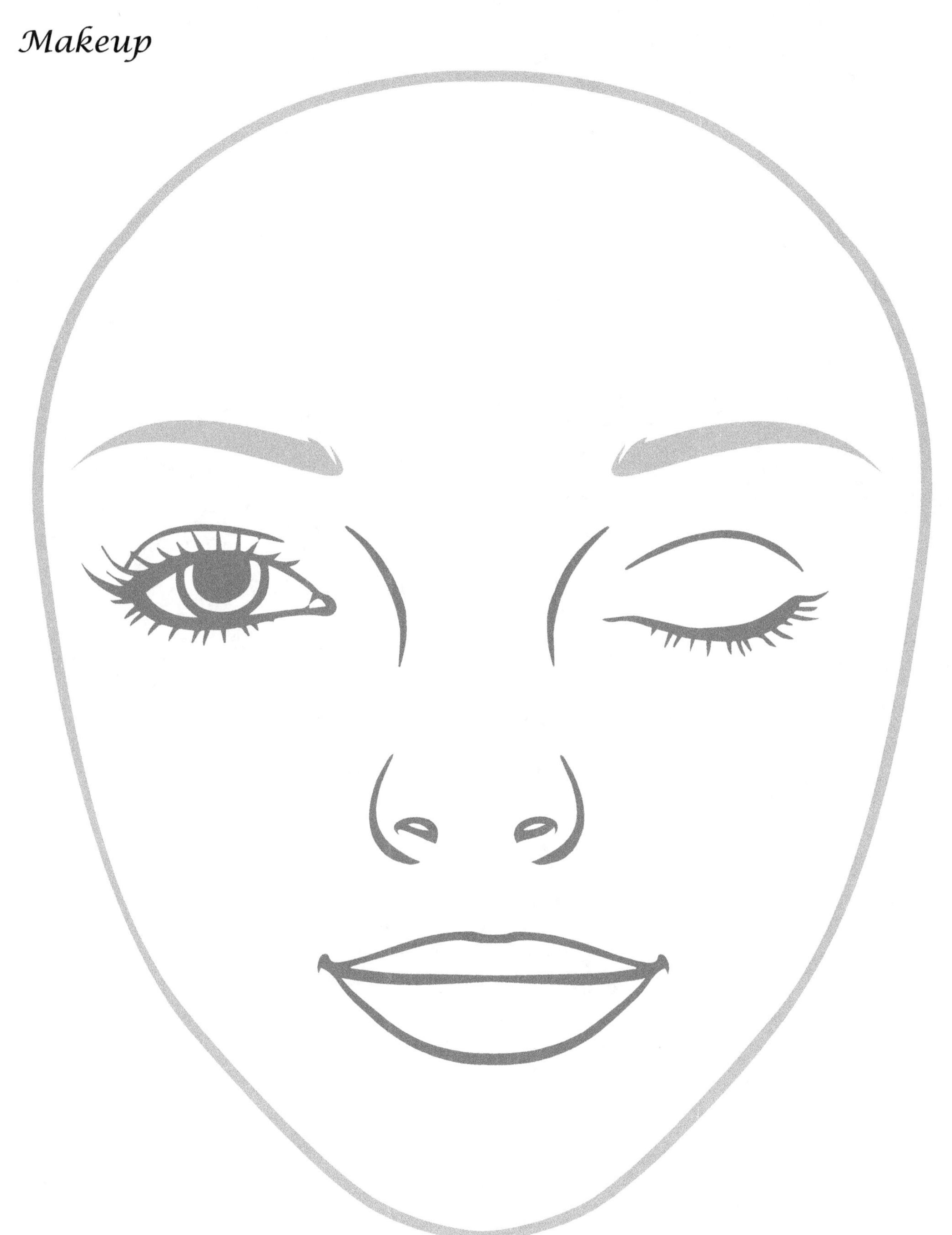
Makeup

Checklist

Checklist